LET'S LOOK AT BODY SYSTEMS!
MIA'S MIGHTY MUSCULAR SYSTEM

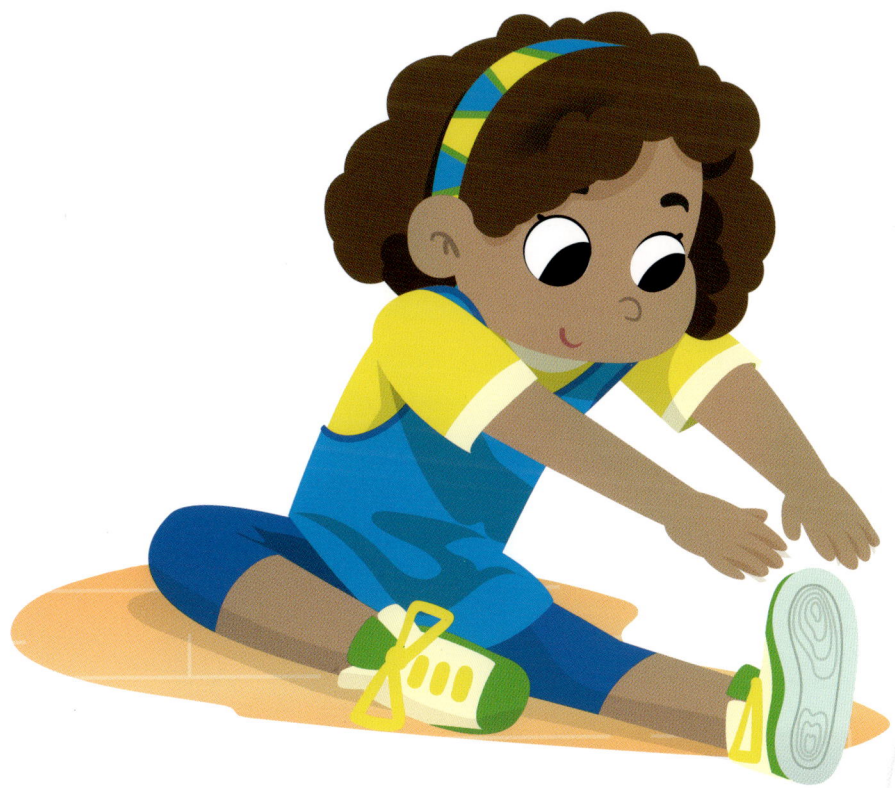

by Mari Schuh
illustrated by Ed Myer

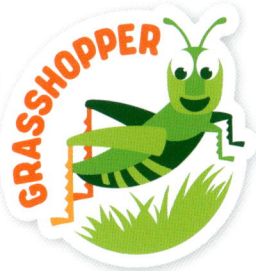

Tools for Parents & Teachers

Grasshopper Books enhance imagination and introduce the earliest readers to fiction with fun storylines and illustrations. The easy-to-read text supports early reading experiences with repetitive sentence patterns and sight words.

Before Reading
- Discuss the cover illustration. What do they see?
- Look at the glossary together. Discuss the words.

Read the Book
- Read the book to the child, or have him or her read independently.
- "Walk" through the book and look at the illustrations. Who is the main character? What is happening in the story?

After Reading
- Prompt the child to think more. Ask: What does your muscular system help you do each day?

Grasshopper Books are published by Jump!
5357 Penn Avenue South
Minneapolis, MN 55419
www.jumplibrary.com

Copyright © 2022 Jump! International copyright reserved in all countries. No part of this book may be reproduced in any form without written permission from the publisher.

Library of Congress Cataloging-in-Publication Data

Names: Schuh, Mari C., 1975- author. | Myer, Ed, illustrator.
Title: Mia's mighty muscular system / by Mari Schuh; illustrated by Ed Myer.
Description: Minneapolis, MN: Jump!, Inc., [2022]
Series: Let's look at body systems! | Includes index.
Audience: Ages 7-10
Identifiers: LCCN 2021038057 (print)
LCCN 2021038058 (ebook)
ISBN 9781636906447 (hardcover)
ISBN 9781636906454 (paperback)
ISBN 9781636906461 (ebook)
Subjects: LCSH: Musculoskeletal system—Juvenile literature.
Muscles—Juvenile literature.
Human physiology—Juvenile literature.
Classification: LCC QP301 .S32 2022 (print)
LCC QP301 (ebook) | DDC 612.7/4—dc23
LC record available at https://lccn.loc.gov/2021038057
LC ebook record available at https://lccn.loc.gov/20210380585

Editor: Jenna Gleisner
Direction and Layout: Anna Peterson
Illustrator: Ed Myer

Printed in the United States of America at Corporate Graphics in North Mankato, Minnesota.

Table of Contents

Moving Muscles..4
Where in the Body?..22
Let's Review!..23
To Learn More...23
Glossary..24
Index...24

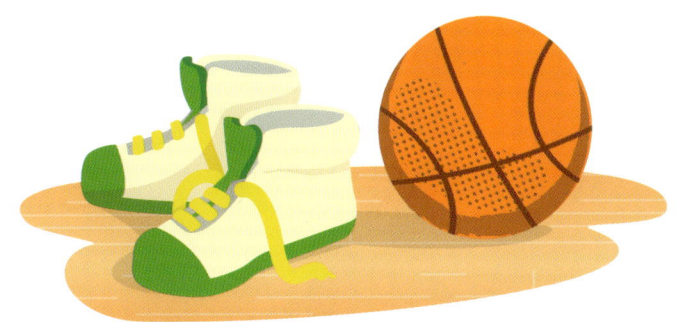

Moving Muscles

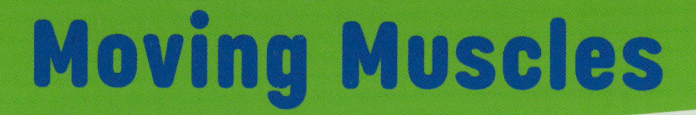

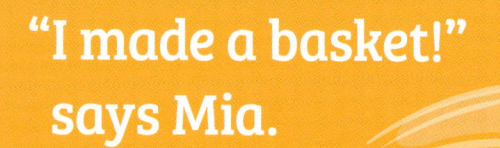

"I made a basket!" says Mia.

"Great job!" her mom says. "Before we play more, let's do some stretching exercises."

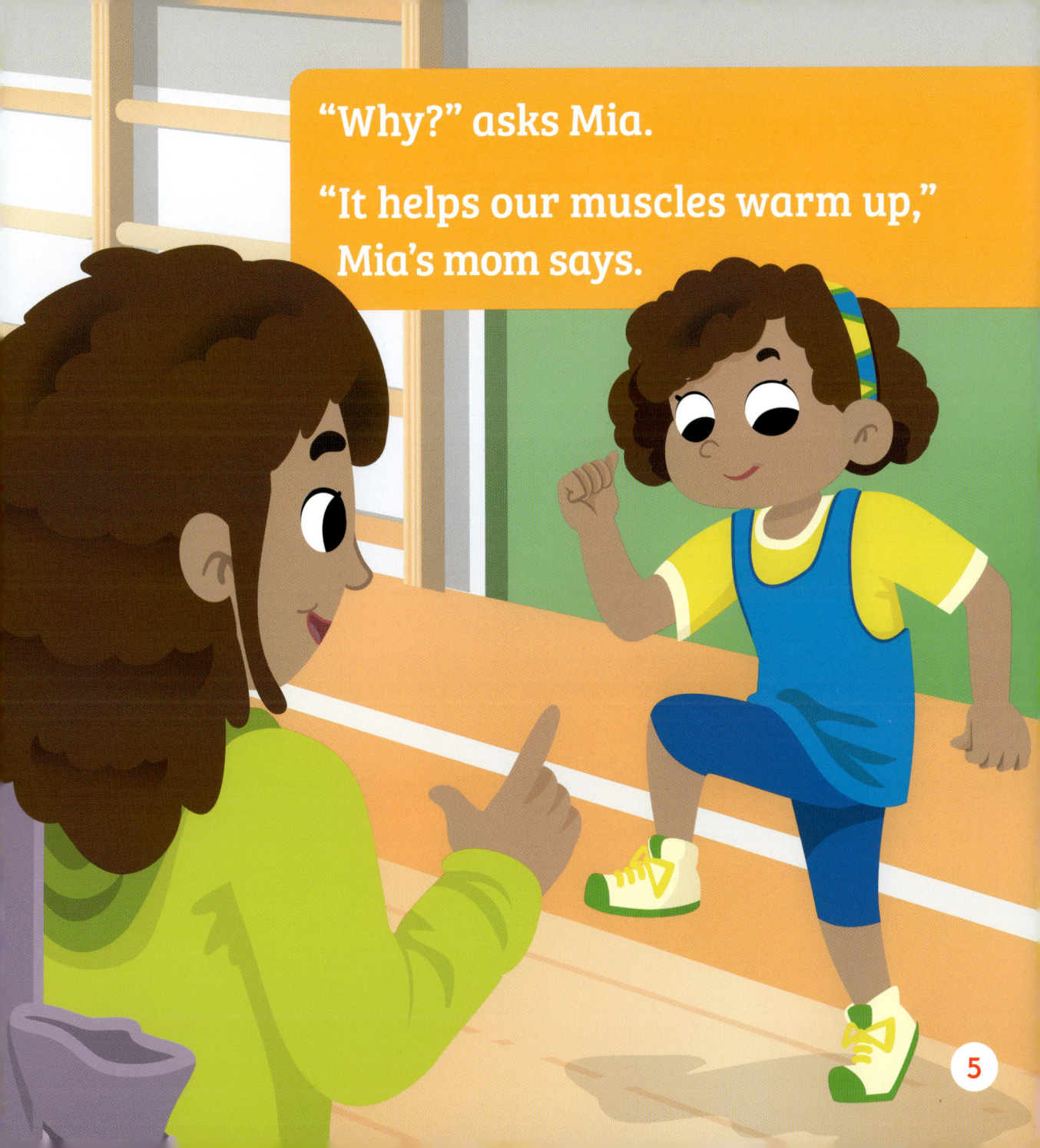

"How do my muscles help me play basketball?" asks Mia.

"Your muscles move your body. They help you shoot and dribble. Your body has more than 600 muscles! Together, they make up your muscular system," says Mia's mom.

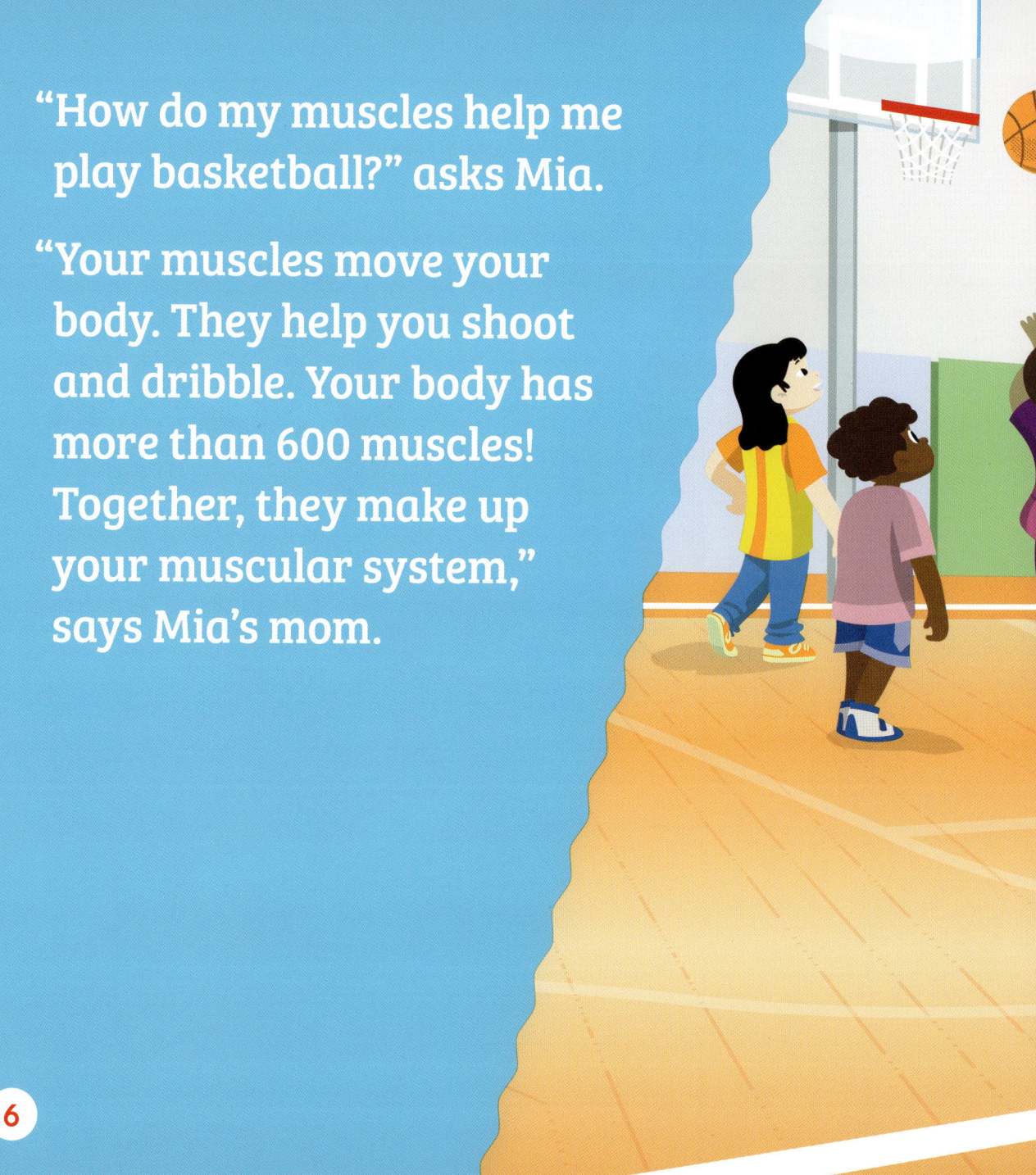

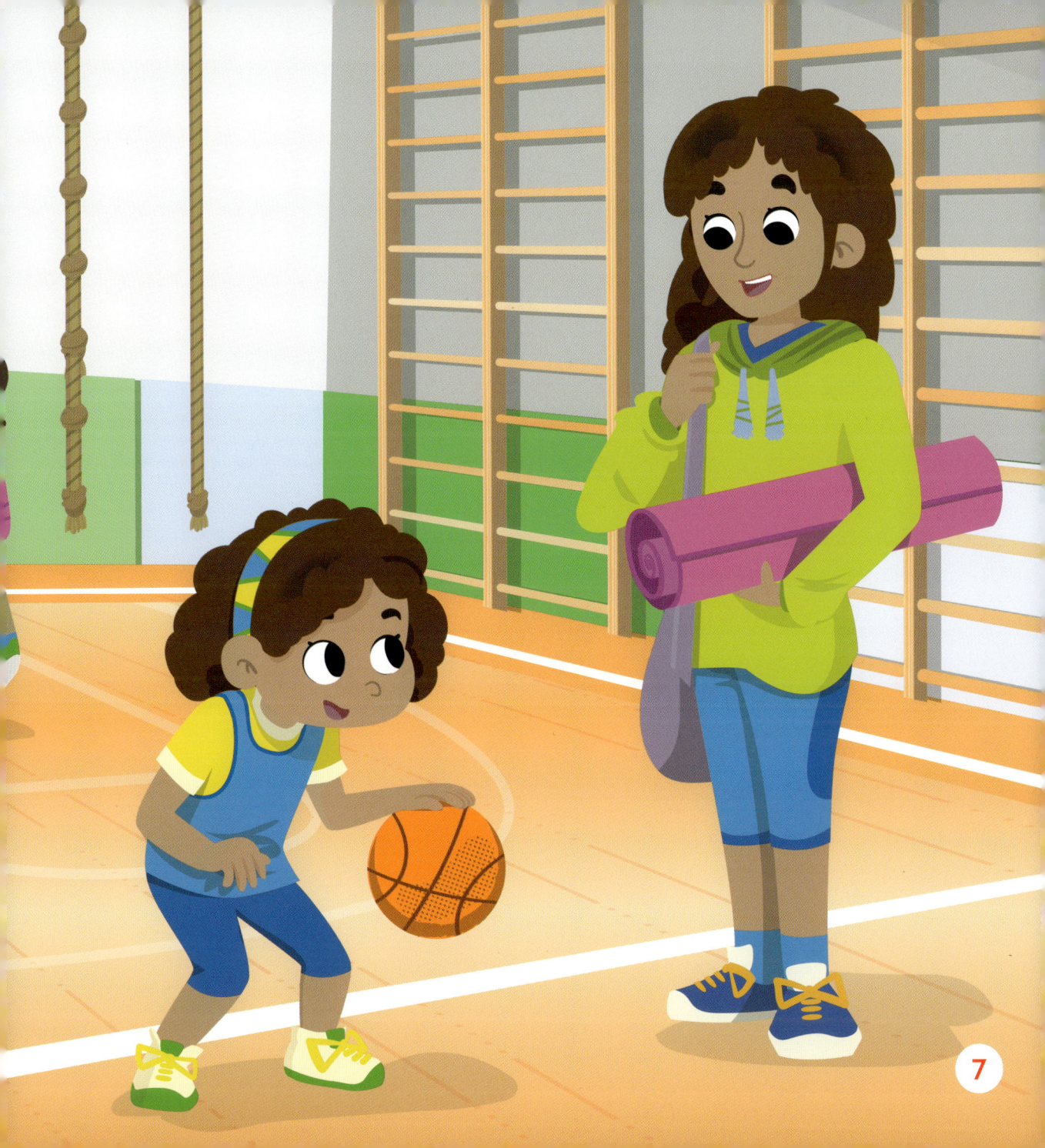

"It's also important to stretch your muscles after exercise. Remember when you strained your calf muscle playing softball last summer?" Mia's mom asks.

"Yeah, I had to miss some games. But ice and rest helped it heal," says Mia.

"That's right!" says Mia's mom.

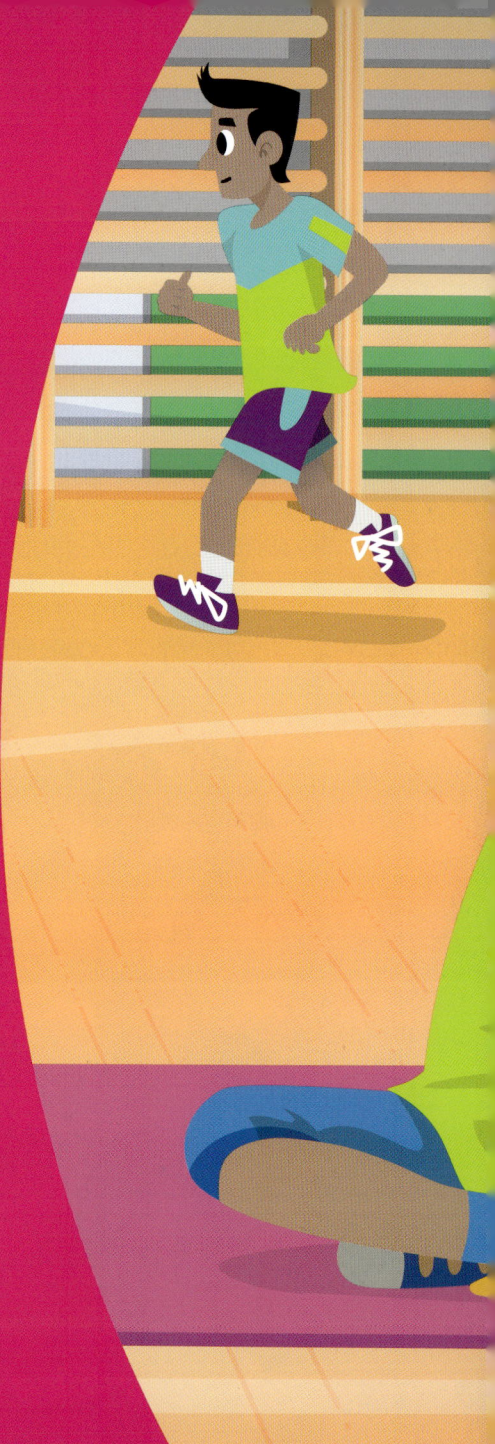

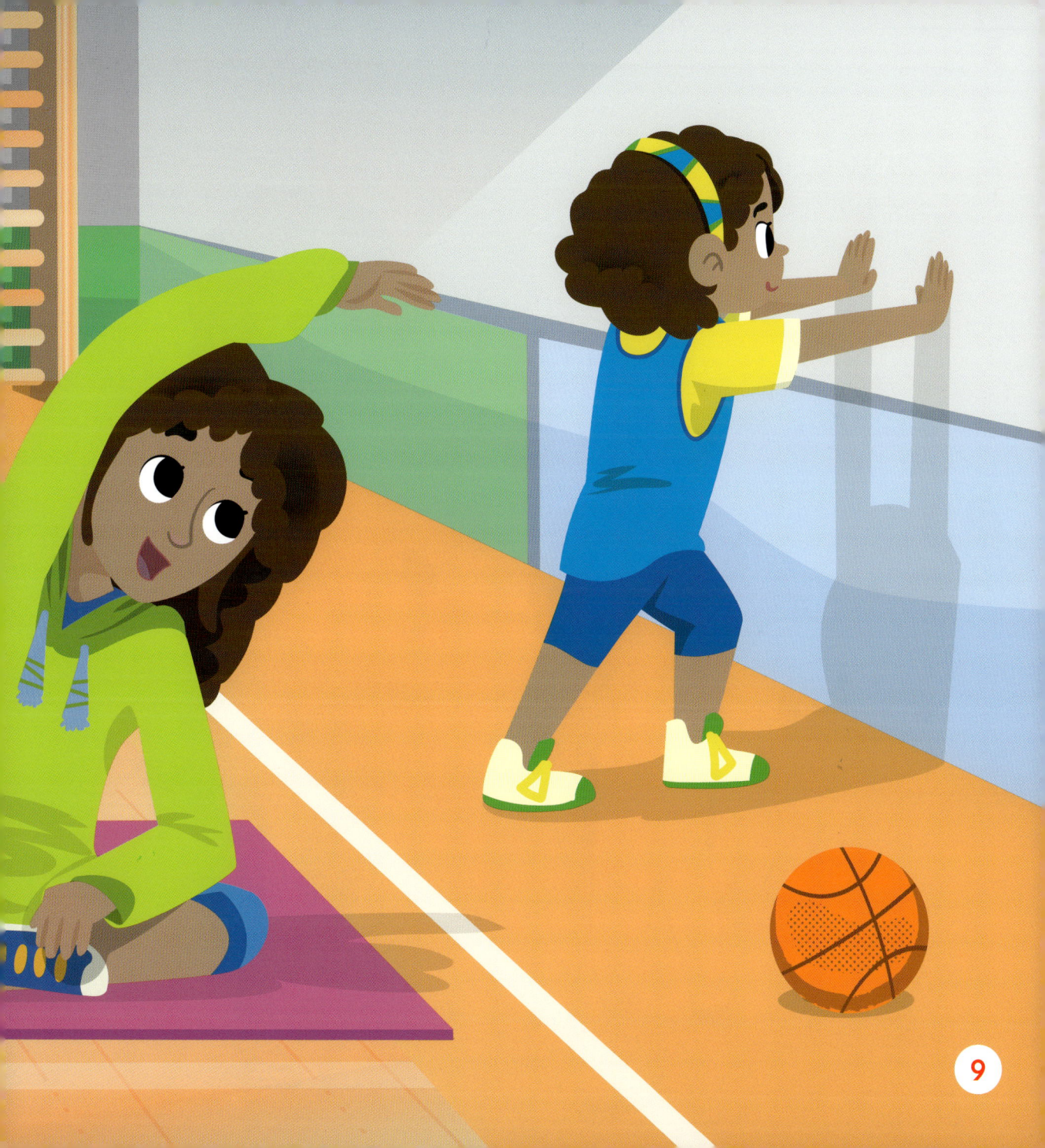

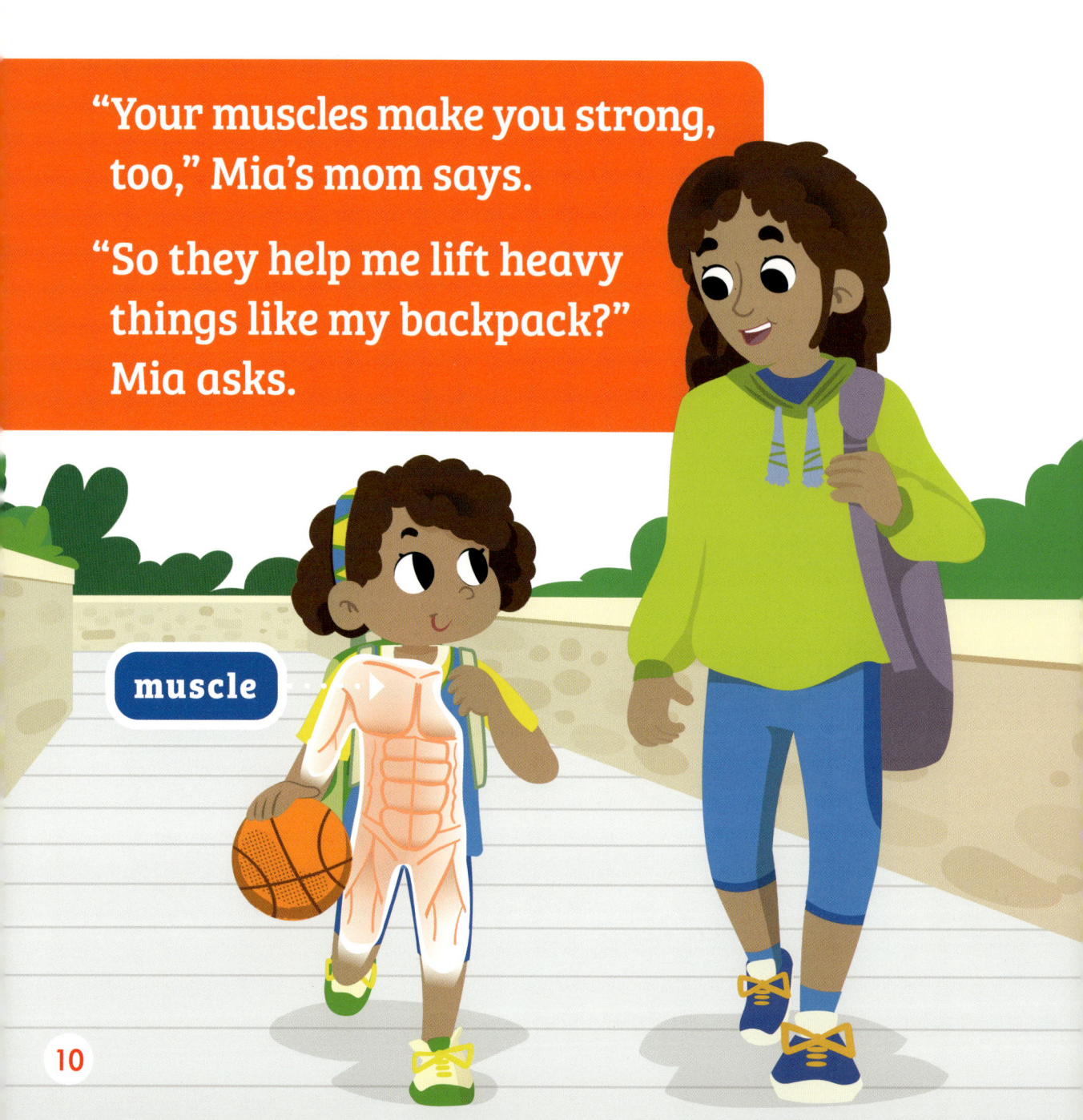

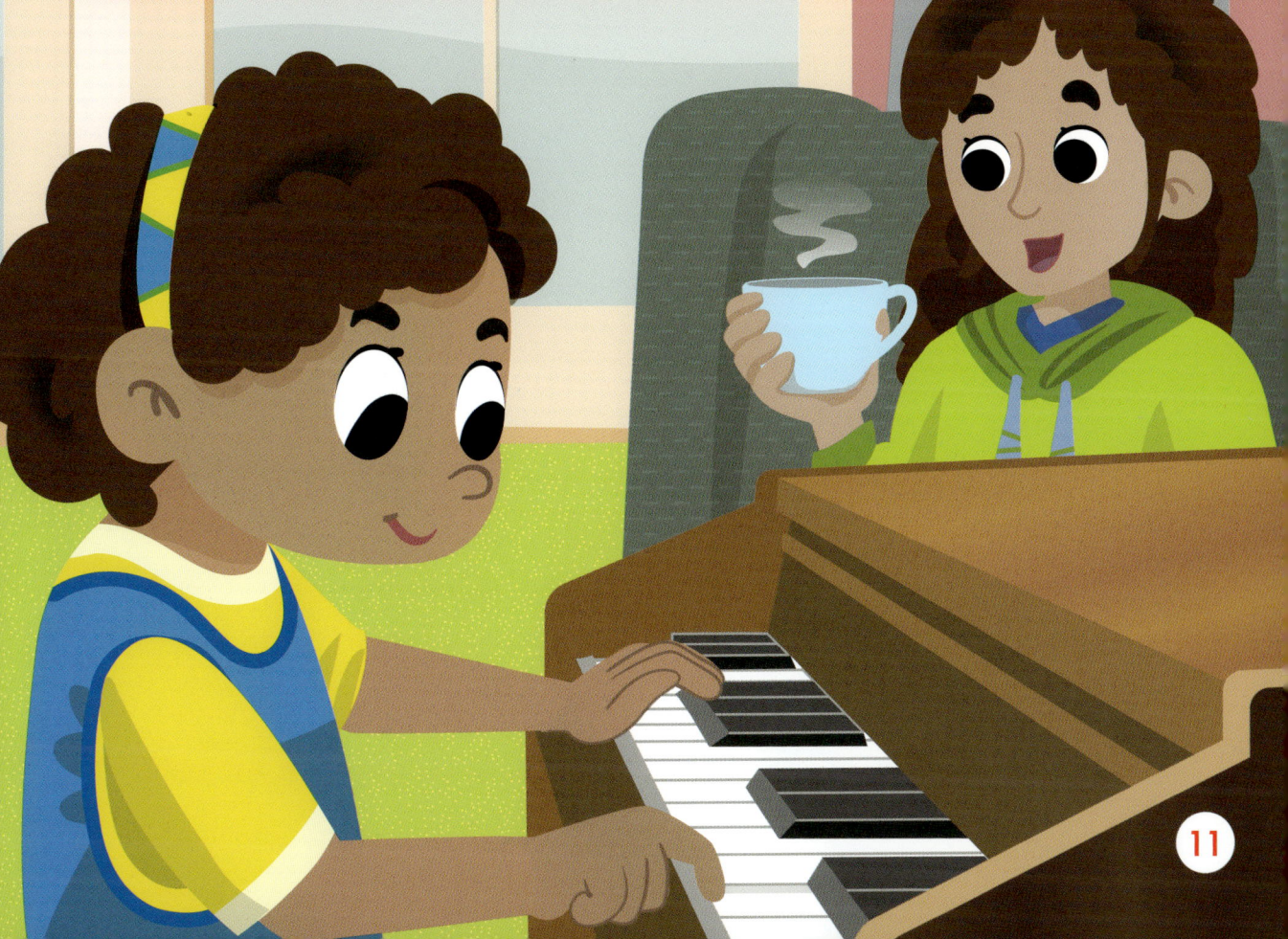

"Yes! But your muscular system does much more than that. Muscles in your hands help you play the piano. Muscles in your face let you blink and smile," Mia's mom explains.

"There are three types of muscles. One is skeletal muscle. Tendons connect these muscles to your bones," Mia's mom explains.

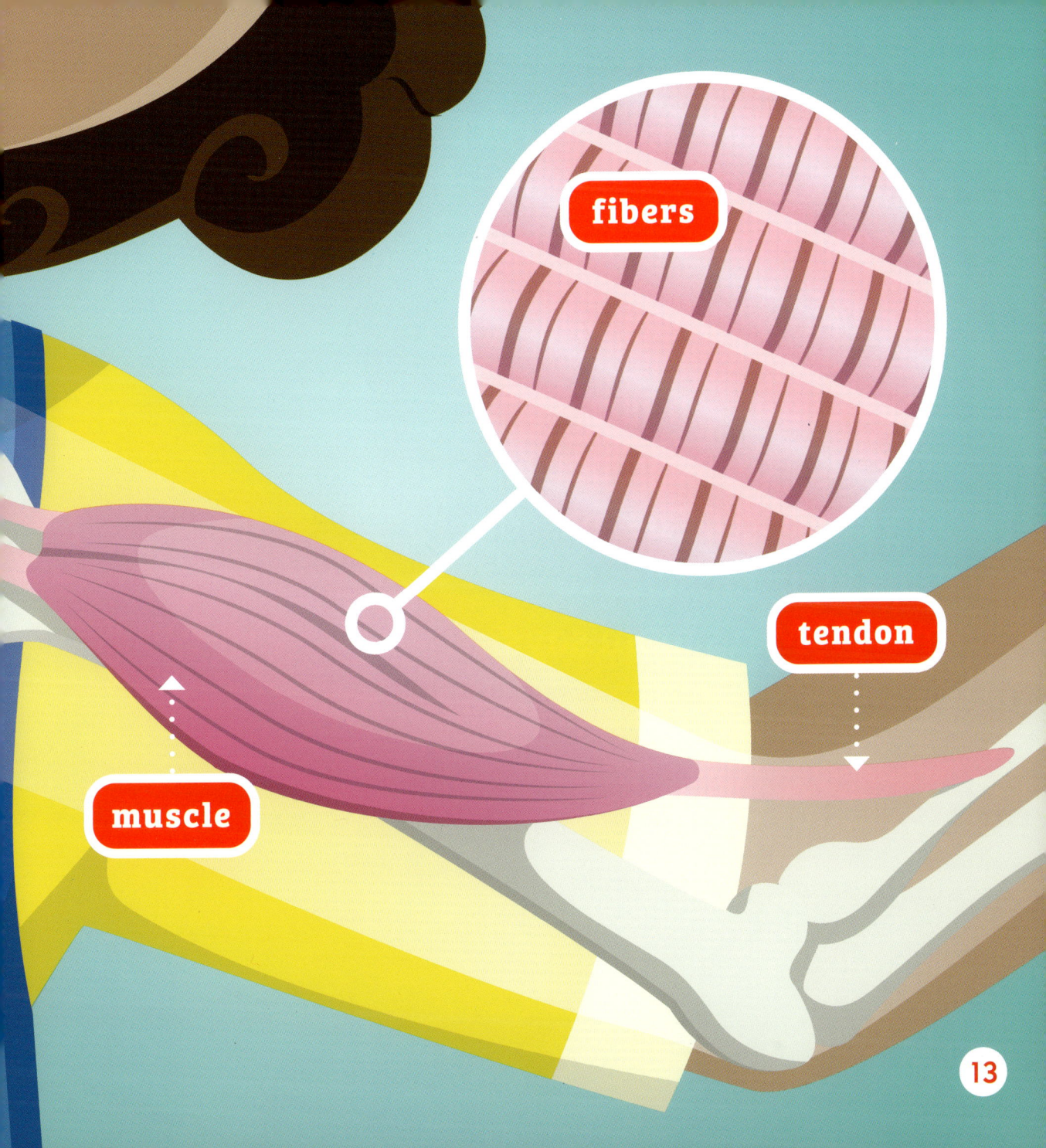

"Skeletal muscles contract and relax to move your bones," Mia's mom says.

"Cool! How?" asks Mia.

"Your brain sends a message through nerves in your body. The message tells your muscles to move!" Mia's mom says.

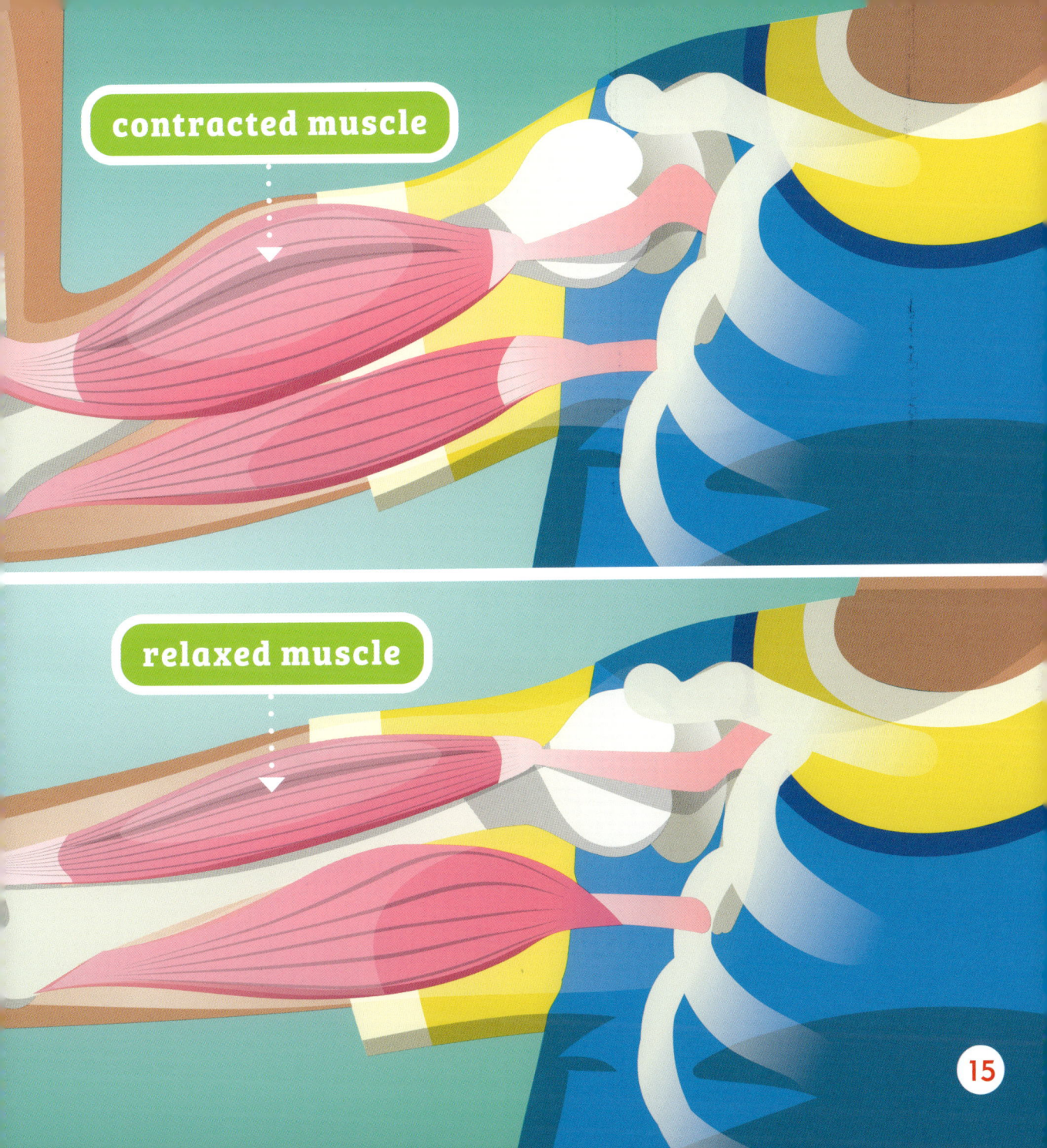

"We also have smooth muscles. These are in hollow organs, such as our stomachs. These muscles work without us thinking about it," her mom says.

"What do they do?" asks Mia.

"They help us breathe and digest food," her mom explains.

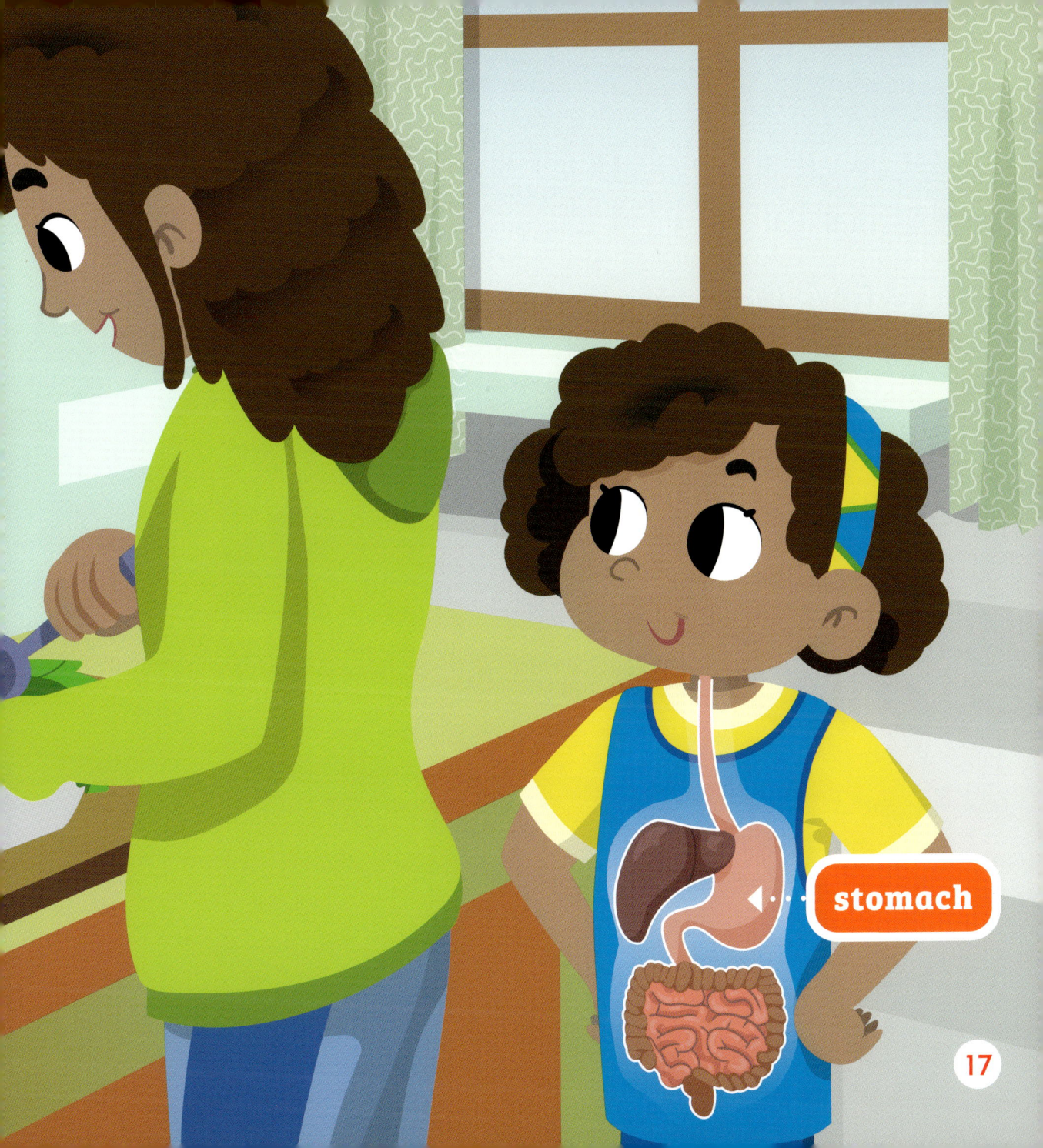

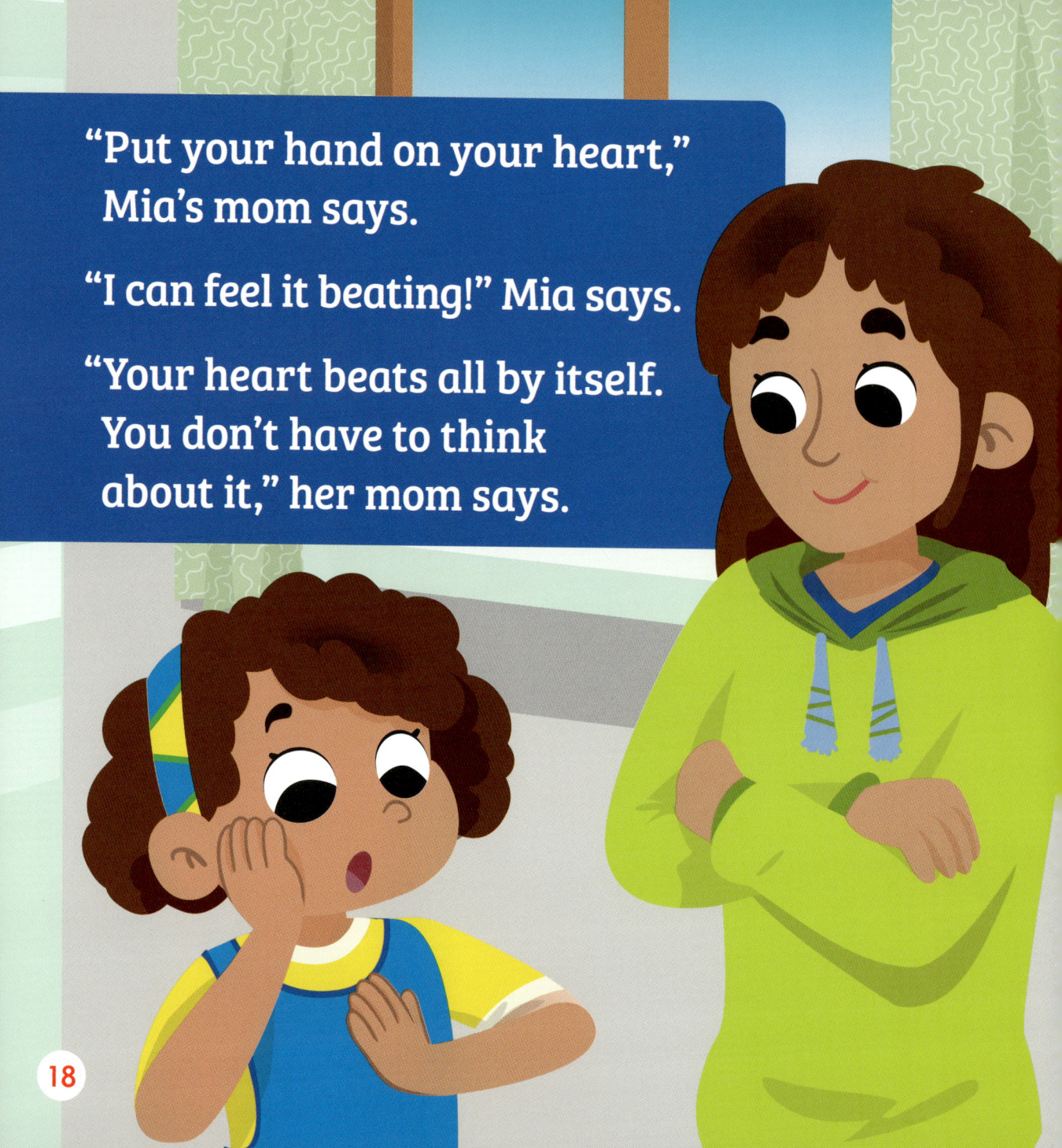

"Your heart is made of muscle, too. It's called cardiac muscle. It contracts to send blood to all parts of your body. Then it relaxes to let blood back into the heart," Mia's mom says.

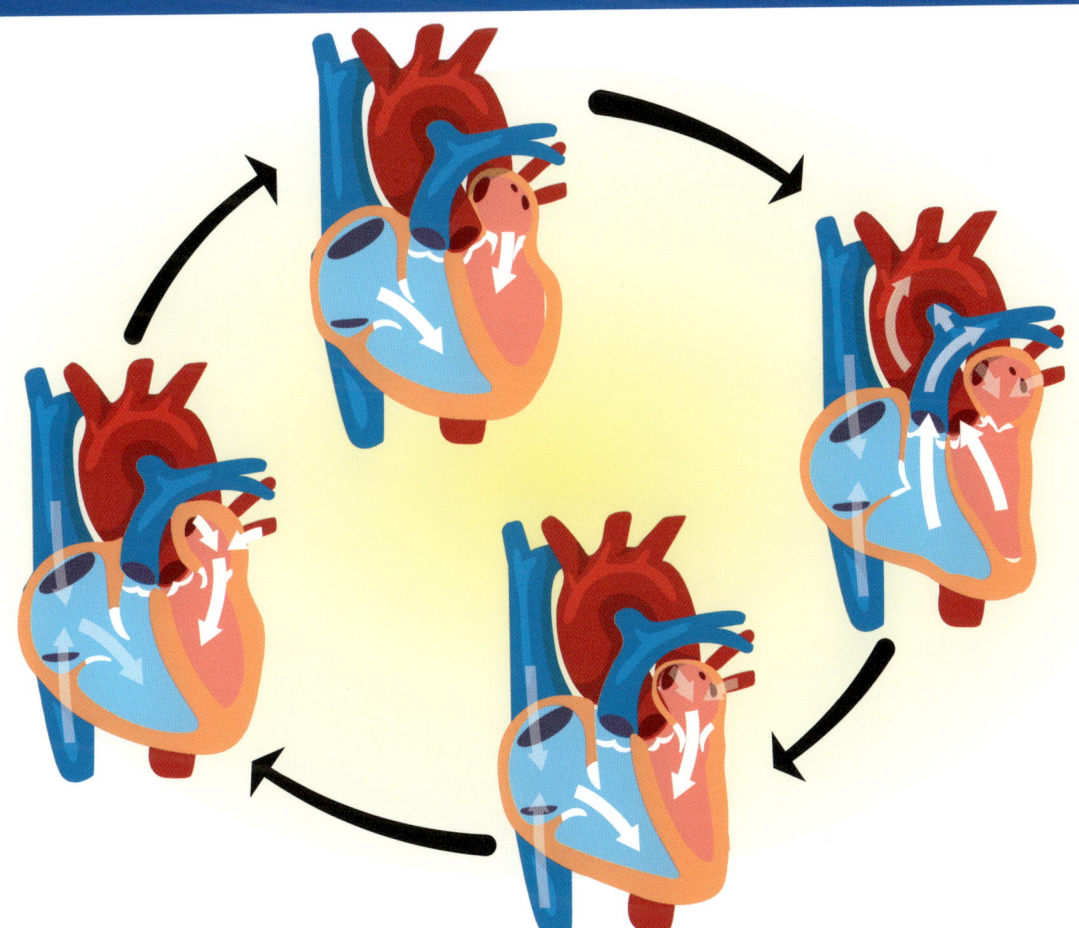

"Eating healthy food helps your muscles grow. Exercise makes them stronger. And when you sleep, your body repairs them!" Mia's mom says.

"That's why my muscles are so strong!" says Mia.

"Good night, mighty Mia," her mom says.

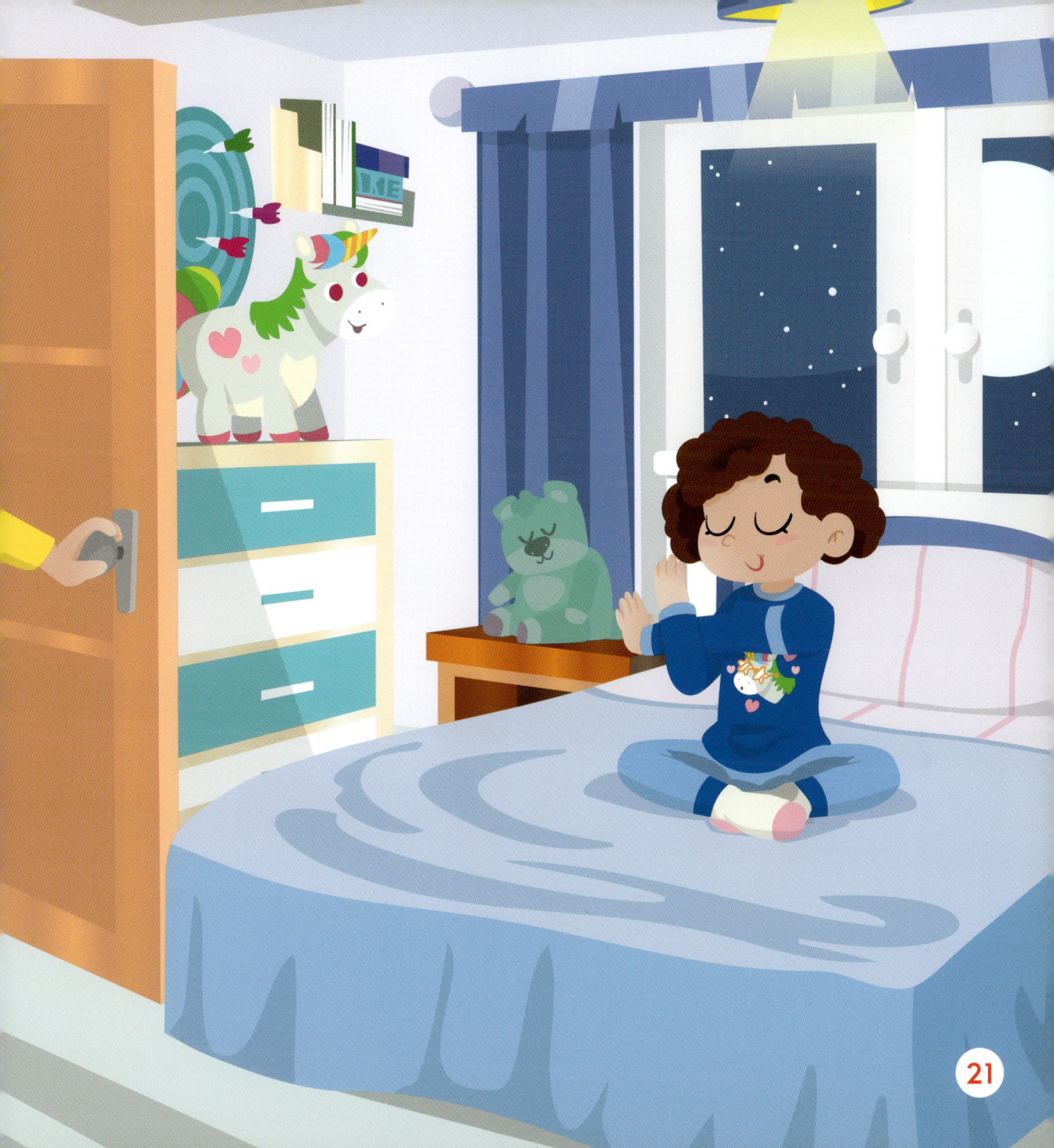

Where in the Body?

What are some of the muscular system's largest muscles called? Take a look!

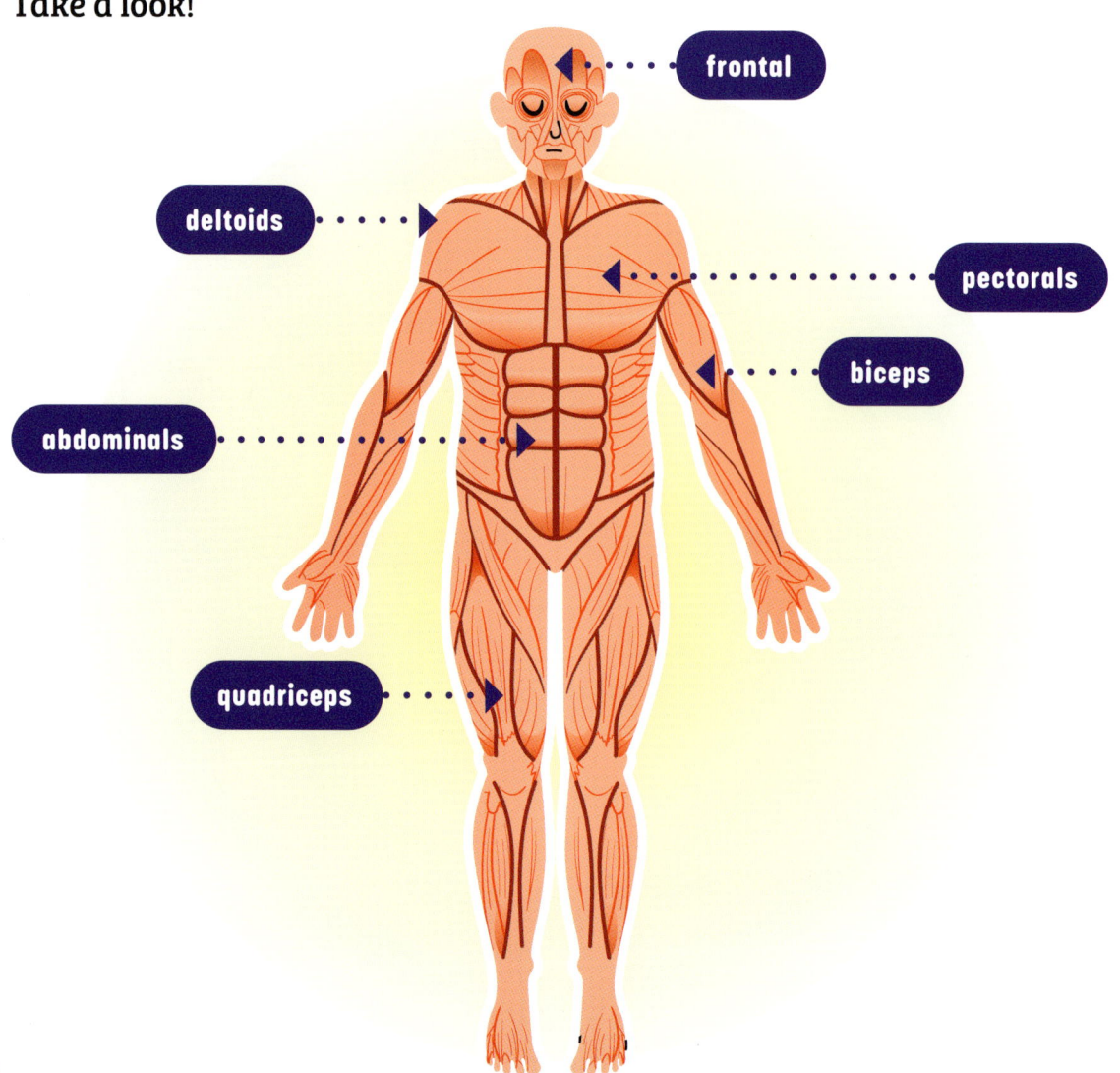

22

Let's Review!

The muscular system is made up of skeletal muscles, smooth muscles, and cardiac muscles. What type of muscle is helping Mia in each of these situations?

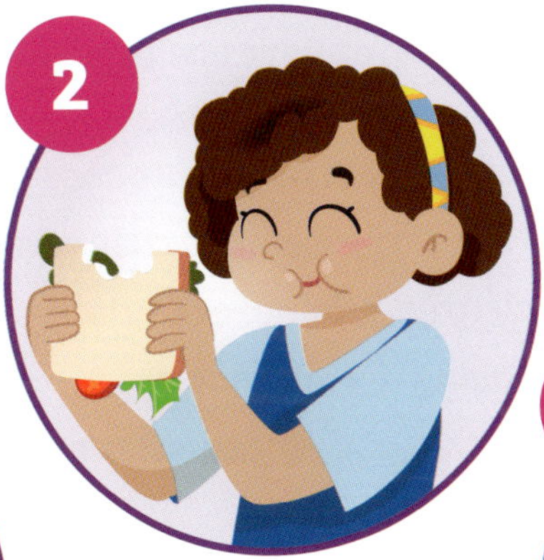

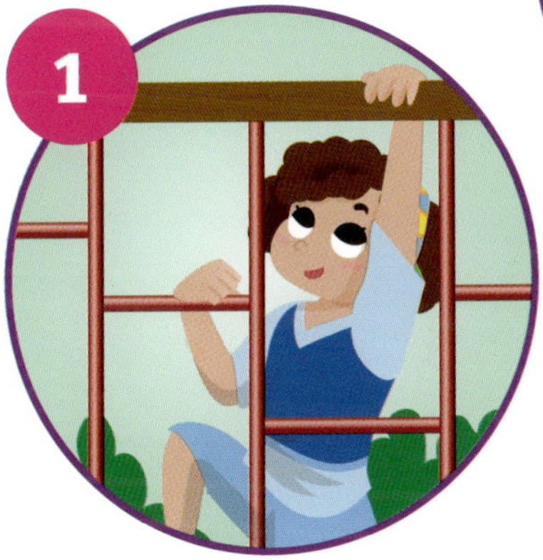

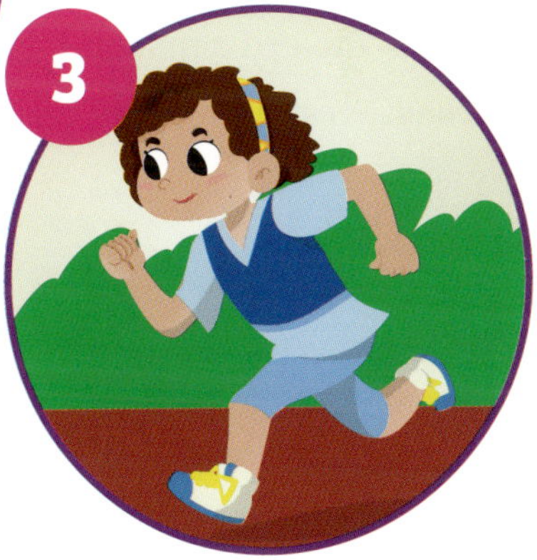

To Learn More

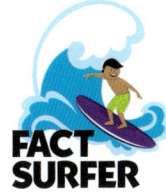

Finding more information is as easy as 1, 2, 3.

1. Go to www.factsurfer.com
2. Enter "**Mia'smightymuscularsystem**" into the search box.
3. Choose your book to see a list of websites.

Let's Review! Answer Key: **1.** skeletal, **2.** smooth, **3.** cardiac.

Glossary

contract: To shorten and tighten.

digest: To break down food in the digestive organs so that it can be absorbed into the blood and used by the body.

hollow organs: Organs that are hollow, or have open space inside, such as the stomach, intestines, and esophagus.

muscles: Tissues in the body that can contract to produce movement.

nerves: Threads of nerve cells that carry messages between the brain and the body.

repairs: Restores, or brings back to an original condition.

strained: Injured a muscle by making it work too hard.

tendons: Stretchy, strong tissues that connect muscles to bones.

Index

blink 11

blood 19

bones 12, 14

breathe 16

cardiac muscle 19

digest 16

heal 8

healthy food 20

heart 18, 19

hollow organs 16

lift 10

nerves 14

repairs 20

skeletal muscle 12, 14

sleep 20

smile 11

smooth muscles 16

strained 8

stretching exercises 4, 8

tendons 12